I0695644

Free Book Offer:

Get How to be a Super Mom For Free

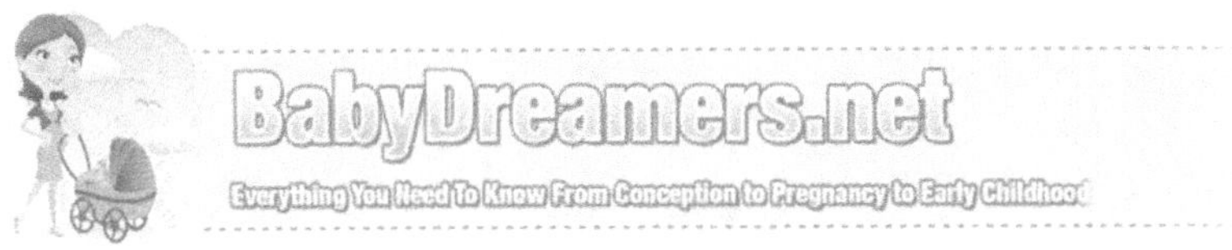

A Short Read is a type of book that is designed to be read in one quick sitting.

These no fluff books are perfect for people who want an overview about a subject in a short period of time.

Table of Contents

The Link Between Stress and Infertility

The link between stress and infertility is a topic that has gained significant attention in recent years. Research has shown that stress levels can have a profound impact on reproductive health and the chances of conceiving. Understanding this connection is crucial for individuals and couples who are trying to start a family.

Studies have revealed that high levels of stress can disrupt the delicate balance of hormones in the body, affecting ovulation in women and sperm production in men. Chronic stress can lead to irregular menstrual cycles, hormonal imbalances, and decreased fertility in women. In men, it can lower sperm count, reduce sperm motility, and increase the risk of erectile dysfunction.

Furthermore, stress can also contribute to the development of reproductive disorders such as polycystic ovary syndrome (PCOS), endometriosis, and uterine fibroids in women. It can disrupt the menstrual cycle, leading to irregular periods, missed periods, or even amenorrhea.

It is important to note that stress does not directly cause infertility, but it can certainly play a role in reducing fertility rates and making it more difficult to conceive. The good news is that there are various stress management techniques and strategies that can help improve reproductive health and increase the chances of successful conception.

Relaxation techniques such as meditation, yoga, and acupuncture have been found to be beneficial in reducing stress levels and enhancing fertility. Regular physical activity and a balanced diet are also important factors in managing stress and optimizing fertility outcomes. Certain foods and supplements, known for their stress-reducing properties, can support reproductive health.

Additionally, seeking professional help in the form of therapies like cognitive-behavioral therapy (CBT) and counseling can be effective in managing stress and improving fertility. Emotional support and mental health care are also crucial during fertility treatments, as stress can significantly impact treatment outcomes.

Alternative medicine, including acupuncture, herbal medicine, and aromatherapy, has gained popularity in reducing stress and improving fertility. These natural approaches can provide additional support to individuals and couples on their fertility journey.

Overall, understanding the link between stress and infertility is essential for those who are trying to conceive. By managing stress levels and seeking appropriate support, individuals and couples can increase their chances of successful conception and improve their overall reproductive health.

Understanding the Stress-Fertility Connection

Examining the scientific research on how stress levels can affect fertility and the chances of getting pregnant.

Stress is an inevitable part of life, and its impact on our health and well-being is well-documented. However, recent studies have shown that stress can also have a significant effect on fertility and the ability to conceive. Understanding the connection between stress and fertility is crucial for individuals and couples who are trying to start a family.

Scientific research has revealed that high levels of stress can disrupt the delicate balance of hormones in the body, leading to reproductive issues. Stress can interfere with the release of reproductive hormones, such as follicle-stimulating hormone (FSH) and luteinizing hormone (LH), which are essential for ovulation and the menstrual cycle in women. In men, stress can negatively impact sperm production and quality.

Studies have shown that women with higher levels of stress are more likely to experience irregular menstrual cycles, hormonal imbalances, and decreased fertility. Chronic stress can disrupt the delicate hormonal balance required for regular ovulation, making it more difficult for women to conceive. Additionally, stress can contribute to conditions like polycystic ovary syndrome (PCOS), endometriosis, and uterine fibroids, further impacting fertility.

In men, chronic stress can lead to lower sperm count, reduced sperm motility, and an increased risk of erectile dysfunction. The quality of sperm can also be affected by stress, with higher levels of stress hormones leading to increased DNA fragmentation and abnormal sperm morphology. These factors can significantly decrease the chances of successful conception.

It is important to note that stress affects individuals differently, and not everyone will experience the same level of impact on their fertility. However, the research consistently indicates that reducing stress levels can improve fertility outcomes. By understanding the stress-fertility connection, individuals and couples can take proactive steps to manage stress and optimize their chances of conceiving.

There are various strategies and techniques available to reduce stress levels and improve reproductive health. These include relaxation techniques such as meditation, yoga, and acupuncture, which have been shown to effectively reduce stress and enhance fertility. Regular physical activity has also been found to play a crucial role in managing stress levels and improving fertility outcomes.

Diet and nutrition also play a significant role in stress reduction and optimizing fertility. A balanced diet that includes specific nutrients, such as antioxidants and omega-3 fatty acids, can help regulate stress hormones and support reproductive health. Certain foods and supplements, known for their stress-reducing properties, can also be beneficial in improving fertility outcomes.

In cases where stress becomes overwhelming and starts to impact daily life, seeking professional help from therapists or counselors specializing in fertility-related stress can be beneficial. Therapies like cognitive-behavioral therapy

(CBT) can provide individuals and couples with effective coping mechanisms and support.

Overall, understanding the stress-fertility connection is crucial for individuals and couples who are trying to conceive. By implementing stress management techniques, seeking emotional support, and making lifestyle changes, individuals can improve their chances of successful conception and navigate the emotional journey of infertility with greater resilience.

The Role of Stress Hormones

The role of stress hormones in the reproductive system is a complex and fascinating topic. One of the key stress hormones that can have a significant impact on fertility is cortisol. Cortisol is released by the body in response to stress and plays a crucial role in the body's stress response.

When cortisol levels are elevated for prolonged periods, it can disrupt the delicate balance of hormones involved in the reproductive system. In women, high levels of cortisol can interfere with the regularity of menstrual cycles, leading to irregular periods or even the absence of menstruation (amenorrhea). This disruption in the menstrual cycle can make it more challenging to predict ovulation and conceive.

In men, chronic stress and high cortisol levels can affect sperm production and quality. Studies have shown that stress can lead to a decrease in sperm count and motility, making it more difficult for sperm to reach and fertilize an egg. Additionally, stress can also increase the risk of erectile dysfunction, further impacting fertility.

The exact mechanisms through which cortisol affects the reproductive system are still being studied, but it is believed that cortisol can interfere with the production of reproductive hormones such as estrogen and progesterone in women, and testosterone in men. These disruptions can have cascading effects on the overall reproductive health and function.

It's important to note that stress hormones like cortisol are a natural part of the body's response to stress, and short-term increases in cortisol levels are not necessarily harmful to fertility. However, chronic and prolonged stress can lead to persistently elevated cortisol levels, which can have detrimental effects on reproductive health.

Managing stress and finding healthy ways to cope with it is crucial for maintaining optimal reproductive function. In the next sections of this article, we will explore various stress management techniques and strategies that can help reduce stress levels and improve fertility outcomes.

Effects of Chronic Stress on Women's Fertility

Chronic stress can have a significant impact on women's fertility, affecting various aspects of their reproductive health. One of the most common effects of long-term stress is the disruption of menstrual cycles. Stress can lead to irregular periods, missed periods, or even the absence of menstruation altogether, a condition known as amenorrhea.

Furthermore, chronic stress can cause hormonal imbalances in women. Stress hormones like cortisol can interfere with the normal production and regulation of reproductive hormones such as estrogen and progesterone. These hormonal imbalances can disrupt the ovulation process, making it more difficult for women to conceive.

In addition to menstrual irregularities and hormonal imbalances, chronic stress can also decrease fertility in women. Studies have shown that high stress levels can negatively impact the quality of eggs released during ovulation. Stress can lead to a decrease in the number of mature eggs available for fertilization, reducing the chances of successful conception.

Moreover, stress can affect the uterine environment, making it less receptive to implantation. The stress response can cause changes in blood flow to the uterus, affecting the development of the uterine lining and reducing the chances of successful embryo implantation.

It is important for women experiencing fertility issues to address and manage their stress levels. By reducing chronic stress, women can improve their menstrual regularity, restore hormonal balance, and enhance their fertility potential. Implementing stress management techniques and seeking support can play a crucial role in optimizing reproductive health and increasing the chances of successful conception.

Effects of Chronic Stress on Men's Fertility

Chronic stress can have a significant impact on men's fertility and reproductive health. When stress levels remain high for extended periods, it can lead to various issues that can affect the quality and quantity of sperm.

One of the primary effects of chronic stress on men's fertility is the decrease in sperm count. High levels of stress hormones, such as cortisol, can interfere with the production of sperm in the testes, leading to a lower sperm count. This can significantly reduce the chances of successful conception.

In addition to lowering sperm count, chronic stress can also reduce sperm motility. Stress hormones can affect the ability of sperm to swim properly, making it more difficult for them to reach and fertilize an egg. This can further decrease the chances of achieving pregnancy.

Furthermore, chronic stress has been linked to an increased risk of erectile dysfunction (ED) in men. Stress can disrupt the hormonal balance in the body, affecting the blood flow to the penis and impairing the ability to achieve and maintain an erection. This can create additional challenges for couples trying to conceive.

It is important for men to recognize the impact of chronic stress on their fertility and take steps to manage stress levels effectively. By reducing stress, men can improve their sperm quality, increase their chances of successful conception, and enhance their overall reproductive health.

The Impact of Stress on Sperm Quality

The impact of stress on sperm quality is a significant concern for men facing fertility issues. Stress can affect various aspects of sperm health, including DNA fragmentation, morphology, and overall quality. When the body is under stress, it releases stress hormones like cortisol, which can disrupt the normal functioning of the reproductive system.

One of the effects of stress on sperm quality is DNA fragmentation. High levels of stress can lead to oxidative stress, causing damage to the DNA within sperm cells. This can result in genetic abnormalities and reduce the chances of successful fertilization and healthy embryo development.

In addition to DNA fragmentation, stress can also affect the morphology or shape of sperm. Studies have shown that men experiencing chronic stress may have a higher percentage of abnormal-shaped sperm, which can impact their ability to swim and fertilize an egg effectively.

Furthermore, stress can have a negative impact on overall sperm health. Chronic stress has been linked to reduced sperm count and motility, making it more difficult for sperm to reach and penetrate the egg for fertilization. Additionally, stress can increase the risk of erectile dysfunction, further complicating the process of conception.

It is important for men to address and manage stress levels when trying to conceive. By reducing stress, men can potentially improve sperm quality and increase their chances of successful fertilization. Implementing stress management techniques, such as exercise, relaxation techniques, and a balanced diet, can help mitigate the negative effects of stress on sperm health.

Psychological Factors and Male Infertility

Infertility can have a significant psychological impact on men, affecting their emotional well-being and overall mental health. The inability to conceive a child can lead to feelings of guilt, shame, and inadequacy, causing stress and anxiety to skyrocket. Men may experience a range of emotions, from frustration and disappointment to sadness and depression.

Stress, in particular, plays a crucial role in male factor infertility. When the body is under chronic stress, it releases stress hormones like cortisol, which can disrupt the delicate balance of the reproductive system. High levels of cortisol can interfere with testosterone production, leading to decreased sperm count and motility.

Furthermore, stress can impact sexual function, contributing to erectile dysfunction and difficulties in achieving or maintaining an erection. The pressure to perform and the constant worry about fertility can create a vicious cycle of stress, further exacerbating the issue.

It is important for men to address the psychological aspects of infertility and seek support when needed. Talking to a therapist or counselor who specializes in fertility-related issues can provide a safe space to express emotions, learn coping strategies, and develop a healthier mindset.

Additionally, engaging in stress-reducing activities such as exercise, meditation, or hobbies can help alleviate anxiety and improve overall well-being.

By addressing the psychological factors associated with male infertility, men can better navigate the emotional journey of fertility struggles and increase their chances of conception.

Stress and Female Reproductive Disorders

Stress can have a significant impact on female reproductive health, potentially contributing to the development or exacerbation of certain conditions. One such condition is polycystic ovary syndrome (PCOS), a hormonal disorder that affects the ovaries and can lead to irregular menstrual cycles, infertility, and other symptoms. Research has shown that stress can worsen the symptoms of PCOS and make it more difficult for women with the condition to conceive.

Endometriosis is another condition that has been linked to stress. This chronic condition occurs when the tissue that normally lines the uterus grows outside of it, causing pain, inflammation, and sometimes fertility problems. While the exact cause of endometriosis is unknown, stress has been identified as a potential contributing factor. Studies have found that women with higher stress levels may be more likely to develop endometriosis or experience more severe symptoms.

Uterine fibroids, non-cancerous growths that develop in the uterus, are also believed to be influenced by stress.

Although the exact relationship between stress and fibroids is not fully understood, research suggests that stress hormones may play a role in their development and growth. Additionally, stress can worsen the symptoms associated with fibroids, such as heavy menstrual bleeding and pelvic pain.

It is important to note that while stress may contribute to the development or progression of these conditions, it is not the sole cause. There are often multiple factors involved, including genetics and hormonal imbalances. However, managing stress levels can still be beneficial for overall reproductive health and may help alleviate some of the symptoms associated with these disorders.

Stress and Menstrual Irregularities

Stress can have a significant impact on the menstrual cycle, causing a range of irregularities and disruptions. When we experience high levels of stress, our bodies release stress hormones like cortisol, which can interfere with the delicate balance of hormones responsible for regulating the menstrual cycle.

One common effect of stress on the menstrual cycle is irregular periods. Stress can cause the length of the menstrual cycle to vary, with periods becoming shorter or longer than usual. This can make it difficult for women to predict when their next period will occur, leading to uncertainty and frustration.

In some cases, stress can even cause missed periods, where menstruation does not occur for one or more cycles. This can be particularly concerning for women who are trying to conceive, as missed periods can make it challenging to track ovulation and determine the most fertile days of the menstrual cycle.

Another potential impact of stress on the menstrual cycle is amenorrhea, which is the absence of menstruation for several months. Chronic stress can disrupt the hormonal signals that trigger ovulation and menstruation, leading to a complete cessation of periods. Amenorrhea can have significant implications for fertility and reproductive health, as it indicates a disruption in the normal functioning of the reproductive system.

It's important to note that stress-related menstrual irregularities are not uncommon and can often be temporary. However, if these irregularities persist or are accompanied by other concerning symptoms, it's essential to consult with a healthcare professional to rule out any underlying medical conditions.

Stress Management Techniques for Improving Fertility

Stress can have a significant impact on fertility and reproductive health. Fortunately, there are several effective stress management techniques that can help improve fertility outcomes. By reducing stress levels, individuals can enhance their reproductive health and increase their chances of conceiving.

Here are some strategies and techniques to consider:

- **1. Relaxation Techniques:** Incorporate relaxation techniques such as meditation, deep breathing exercises, and progressive muscle relaxation into your daily routine. These practices can help calm the mind, reduce stress, and promote overall well-being.
- **2. Exercise:** Engage in regular physical activity to release endorphins, boost mood, and reduce stress levels. Aim for at least 30 minutes of moderate-intensity exercise most days of the week.
- **3. Healthy Diet:** Maintain a balanced diet rich in fruits, vegetables, whole grains, lean proteins, and healthy fats. Avoid excessive caffeine, alcohol, and processed foods, as they can contribute to stress and hormonal imbalances.
- **4. Adequate Sleep:** Prioritize getting enough sleep each night. Aim for 7-9 hours of uninterrupted sleep to support hormonal balance and reduce stress levels.
- **5. Time Management:** Develop effective time management skills to reduce feelings of overwhelm and stress. Prioritize tasks, delegate

when possible, and create a schedule that allows for relaxation and self-care.

- **6. Support System:** Seek support from loved ones, friends, or support groups. Sharing your feelings and experiences with others who understand can provide emotional relief and reduce stress.
- **7. Mindfulness:** Practice mindfulness techniques, such as being present in the moment and focusing on positive thoughts and affirmations. Mindfulness can help reduce stress and improve overall well-being.

Remember, stress management is a personal journey, and what works for one person may not work for another. It's essential to find the techniques that resonate with you and incorporate them into your daily routine. By reducing stress levels, you can create a more conducive environment for fertility and increase your chances of conceiving.

Relaxation Techniques and Fertility

When it comes to managing stress and improving fertility, relaxation techniques can play a vital role. Techniques such as meditation, yoga, and acupuncture have been shown to reduce stress levels and enhance fertility outcomes.

Meditation:

Meditation is a practice that involves focusing the mind and achieving a state of deep relaxation. It can help reduce stress and anxiety, promote emotional well-being, and improve overall fertility. By incorporating meditation into your daily routine, you can create a sense of calm and balance, which can positively impact your reproductive health.

Yoga:

Yoga combines physical postures, breathing exercises, and meditation to promote relaxation and improve overall well-being. It can help reduce stress levels, increase blood flow to the reproductive organs, and balance hormone levels. By practicing yoga regularly, you can create a harmonious environment for conception and support your fertility journey.

Acupuncture:

Acupuncture is an ancient Chinese therapy that involves the insertion of thin needles into specific points on the body. It is believed to restore the flow of energy, or Qi, and promote overall well-being. Acupuncture has been shown to reduce stress, regulate hormone levels, and improve blood flow to the reproductive organs. By incorporating acupuncture into your fertility treatment plan, you can enhance your chances of conception.

Overall, relaxation techniques such as meditation, yoga, and acupuncture offer a holistic approach to managing stress and improving fertility. By incorporating these practices into your daily routine, you can create a sense of calm, reduce stress levels, and enhance your reproductive health.

Impact of Exercise on Stress and Fertility

The impact of exercise on stress and fertility is significant. Regular physical activity plays a crucial role in managing stress levels and improving fertility outcomes. Engaging in exercise not only helps to reduce stress but also promotes overall well-being and reproductive health.

When we exercise, our bodies release endorphins, which are natural mood boosters. These endorphins help to alleviate stress and promote a sense of well-being. Regular exercise also helps to reduce the levels of stress hormones, such as cortisol, in our bodies. By reducing cortisol levels, exercise can help to regulate the reproductive system and improve fertility.

In addition to reducing stress, exercise also has a positive impact on fertility. It helps to improve blood circulation, which is essential for reproductive health. Increased blood flow to the reproductive organs can enhance the chances of successful conception. Exercise also helps to maintain a healthy weight, which is crucial for fertility. Being overweight or underweight can negatively affect fertility, and regular exercise can help to maintain a healthy body weight.

It is important to note that when it comes to exercise and fertility, moderation is key. Overexercising or engaging in intense workouts can have adverse effects on fertility. It is recommended to engage in moderate-intensity exercises, such as brisk walking, swimming, or cycling, for about 30 minutes a day, most days of the week.

It is also essential to listen to your body and make adjustments as needed. If you are undergoing fertility treatments or have specific medical conditions, it is advisable to consult with your healthcare provider before starting or modifying an exercise routine.

In conclusion, regular exercise is not only beneficial for managing stress but also plays a crucial role in improving fertility outcomes. By incorporating moderate-intensity exercises into your daily routine, you can reduce stress levels, promote overall well-being, and enhance your chances of conceiving.

Diet and Nutrition for Stress Reduction

When it comes to managing stress and optimizing fertility, diet and nutrition play a crucial role. A balanced diet rich in essential nutrients can help reduce stress levels and support reproductive health. Here are some key considerations for incorporating a stress-reducing diet into your lifestyle:

- **Load up on fruits and vegetables:** These colorful and nutrient-rich foods are packed with antioxidants, vitamins, and minerals that help combat stress and promote overall well-being. Aim for a variety of fruits and vegetables to ensure you're getting a wide range of nutrients.
- **Include whole grains:** Whole grains like brown rice, quinoa, and oats are not only a great source of energy but also contain fiber and B vitamins

that support the nervous system and help regulate mood.

- **Choose lean proteins:** Opt for lean sources of protein such as poultry, fish, beans, and tofu. Protein helps stabilize blood sugar levels and provides amino acids that are essential for neurotransmitter production, which can positively impact mood and stress levels.
- **Don't forget healthy fats:** Incorporate sources of healthy fats like avocados, nuts, seeds, and olive oil into your diet. These fats help reduce inflammation, support brain health, and provide a steady source of energy.

In addition to these general guidelines, there are specific nutrients that have been shown to have stress-reducing and fertility-boosting properties:

Nutrient	Sources
Omega-3 fatty acids	Fatty fish (salmon, sardines), walnuts, flaxseeds, chia seeds
B vitamins	Whole grains, leafy greens, legumes, eggs, nuts
Vitamin C	Citrus fruits, strawberries, kiwi, bell peppers
Magnesium	Dark chocolate, spinach, almonds, pumpkin seeds

Zinc   Oysters, beef, poultry, beans, nuts

It's important to note that while a healthy diet can support stress reduction and fertility, it's not a magic solution. It should be combined with other stress management techniques and medical guidance if needed. Consult with a healthcare professional or a registered dietitian to create a personalized diet plan that suits your specific needs and goals.

Stress-Reducing Foods and Supplements

When it comes to managing stress and supporting reproductive health, certain foods and supplements can play a crucial role. These stress-reducing foods and supplements not only help regulate stress hormones but also provide essential nutrients that support overall reproductive health.

One of the key nutrients for stress reduction is magnesium. Magnesium-rich foods like leafy greens, nuts, and seeds can help relax the muscles and promote a sense of calm. Additionally, supplements like magnesium citrate or magnesium glycinate can be beneficial in regulating stress hormones and improving fertility outcomes.

Omega-3 fatty acids are another important component of stress-reducing foods. These healthy fats can be found in fatty fish like salmon, sardines, and mackerel. Omega-3 fatty acids have been shown to reduce inflammation and support brain health, which can help alleviate stress and improve reproductive function.

Probiotics, commonly found in fermented foods like yogurt, kefir, and sauerkraut, can also have a positive impact on stress levels. The gut-brain connection is well-established, and maintaining a healthy gut microbiome through probiotic-rich foods or supplements can help regulate stress responses and support reproductive health.

In addition to these foods, certain supplements can provide targeted support for stress reduction and reproductive health. Adaptogenic herbs like ashwagandha, rhodiola, and holy basil have been used for centuries to help the body adapt to stress and promote hormonal balance. These herbs can be taken in supplement form or consumed as teas.

It's important to note that while stress-reducing foods and supplements can be beneficial, they should not replace a balanced diet and a healthy lifestyle. It's always best to consult with a healthcare professional or a registered dietitian before making any significant changes to your diet or starting any new supplements.

The Gut-Brain Axis and Stress

The Gut-Brain Axis and Stress

The gut-brain axis is a complex communication network that connects the gut and the brain. It involves bidirectional communication between the central nervous system and the enteric nervous system, which is responsible for regulating the function of the gastrointestinal tract. Recent research has shown that this gut-brain connection plays a crucial role in various aspects of health, including stress and fertility.

Stress can have a profound impact on gut health, disrupting the balance of beneficial bacteria in the gut and compromising the integrity of the intestinal lining. This disruption can lead to a condition called "leaky gut," where the gut becomes more permeable, allowing toxins and harmful substances to enter the bloodstream. These changes in gut health can trigger an inflammatory response in the body and contribute to increased stress levels.

Furthermore, the gut microbiota, which refers to the community of microorganisms residing in the gut, plays a crucial role in regulating stress and emotional well-being. The gut microbiota produces various neurotransmitters and hormones that influence mood, including serotonin, dopamine, and gamma-aminobutyric acid (GABA). Imbalances in the gut microbiota have been linked to mental health disorders such as anxiety and depression, which are often associated with increased stress levels.

Interestingly, emerging evidence suggests that improving gut health through diet, lifestyle changes, and targeted supplementation can help reduce stress levels and enhance fertility outcomes. By restoring the balance of beneficial bacteria in the gut and reducing inflammation, individuals may experience a reduction in stress and an improvement in reproductive health.

One way to support gut health is through a balanced and nutritious diet. Consuming a variety of fiber-rich foods, such as fruits, vegetables, whole grains, and legumes, can promote a healthy gut microbiota. Additionally, incorporating fermented foods like yogurt, sauerkraut, and kimchi can introduce beneficial probiotic bacteria into the gut.

Another approach to improving gut health and reducing stress is through the use of targeted supplements. Probiotics, which are live bacteria and yeasts that are beneficial for gut health, can help restore the balance of the gut microbiota. Additionally, certain herbs and botanicals, such as ashwagandha and chamomile, have been traditionally used to support stress reduction and promote overall well-being.

In conclusion, the gut-brain axis plays a crucial role in the connection between gut health, stress, and fertility. By improving gut health through dietary changes, targeted supplementation, and stress reduction techniques, individuals may be able to reduce stress levels and enhance their chances of conceiving. It is important to consult with healthcare professionals or fertility specialists to develop a personalized plan that addresses individual needs and optimizes reproductive health.

Therapies and Counseling for Stress Management

Therapies and counseling play a crucial role in managing stress and improving fertility outcomes. One effective therapy is cognitive-behavioral therapy (CBT), which focuses on identifying and changing negative thought patterns and behaviors that contribute to stress. By addressing these patterns, CBT helps individuals develop healthier coping mechanisms and reduce stress levels.

Counseling, on the other hand, provides a safe and supportive space for individuals and couples to explore their emotions and concerns related to fertility issues. It allows them to express their feelings, gain insight into their experiences, and develop strategies for managing stress. Counseling can be particularly beneficial for couples, as it helps improve communication, strengthen the partnership, and navigate the emotional challenges of infertility together.

In addition to CBT and counseling, other therapeutic approaches such as mindfulness-based stress reduction (MBSR) and acceptance and commitment therapy (ACT) have also shown promise in managing stress and enhancing fertility. These therapies focus on cultivating mindfulness, acceptance, and self-compassion, which can help individuals cope with the emotional roller coaster of infertility.

It's important to note that therapies and counseling should be tailored to individual needs and preferences. Some individuals may find group therapy or support groups helpful, as they provide a sense of community and validation. Others may benefit from individual therapy or couples counseling to address specific concerns and relationship dynamics.

Overall, therapies and counseling offer valuable tools and support for managing stress during the fertility journey. They provide individuals and couples with the skills and strategies needed to cope with the emotional challenges of infertility, improve overall well-being, and increase the chances of successful conception.

Supporting Emotional Well-being During Fertility Treatment

The journey of fertility treatment can be emotionally challenging for individuals and couples. It is essential to recognize the importance of emotional support and mental health care during this time. The impact of stress on treatment outcomes cannot be overlooked, as stress can have a significant influence on fertility.

Emotional well-being plays a crucial role in fertility treatment. The stress and anxiety that often accompany the process can affect hormonal balance, disrupt ovulation, and even impact the success of assisted reproductive technologies (ART) such as in vitro fertilization (IVF). Therefore, it is essential to prioritize emotional support and mental health care throughout the fertility treatment journey.

One way to support emotional well-being during fertility treatment is to seek professional help. Therapists and counselors who specialize in infertility can provide guidance and support, helping individuals and couples navigate the emotional challenges that arise. These professionals can help individuals develop coping strategies, manage stress, and address any underlying emotional issues that may be affecting fertility.

Support groups and online communities can also be invaluable sources of emotional support. Connecting with others who are going through similar experiences can reduce feelings of isolation and provide a sense of belonging. Sharing experiences, insights, and coping strategies can be incredibly empowering and can help individuals and couples feel less alone on their fertility journey.

Communication and partner support are also vital components of supporting emotional well-being during fertility treatment. Open and honest communication with your partner can help alleviate stress and strengthen the partnership. Sharing fears, hopes, and concerns can foster a sense of togetherness and provide a support system for both individuals.

Additionally, self-care should not be overlooked during this challenging time. Engaging in activities that promote relaxation and reduce stress can have a positive impact on emotional well-being and fertility outcomes. This could include practices such as meditation, yoga, journaling, or engaging in hobbies that bring joy and fulfillment.

Overall, supporting emotional well-being during fertility treatment is crucial for both individuals and couples. Recognizing the impact of stress on treatment outcomes and prioritizing emotional support, mental health care, and self-care can help individuals navigate the challenges of fertility treatment with resilience and hope.

Alternative Medicine and Stress Reduction

Alternative medicine offers a holistic approach to reducing stress and improving fertility. These therapies focus on addressing the mind, body, and spirit to promote overall well-being and enhance reproductive health. Alternative therapies such as acupuncture, herbal medicine, and aromatherapy have gained popularity for their potential benefits in reducing stress levels and supporting fertility.

Acupuncture: Acupuncture is an ancient Chinese practice that involves the insertion of thin needles into specific points on the body. It is believed to help restore balance and promote the flow of energy, known as Qi. Acupuncture has been shown to reduce stress and anxiety levels, which can have a positive impact on fertility. It may also help regulate hormonal imbalances and improve blood flow to the reproductive organs, increasing the chances of conception.

Herbal Medicine: Herbal medicine utilizes the healing properties of plants to support the body's natural functions. Certain herbs have been traditionally used to reduce stress and promote relaxation, such as chamomile, lavender, and passionflower. Herbal remedies can help regulate hormone levels, improve reproductive health, and reduce the negative effects of chronic stress on fertility.

Aromatherapy: Aromatherapy involves the use of essential oils derived from plants to promote relaxation and reduce stress. Essential oils like lavender, rose, and ylang-ylang can be used in diffusers, baths, or massage oils to create a calming environment and alleviate anxiety. Aromatherapy can help reduce stress levels, improve sleep quality, and enhance overall well-being, which can positively impact fertility.

While alternative therapies can be beneficial in reducing stress and improving fertility, it is important to consult with a qualified practitioner and discuss any potential risks or interactions with other medications or treatments. These therapies should be used as complementary approaches alongside conventional medical care for the best results.

Acupuncture and Stress Reduction

Acupuncture is an ancient Chinese medical practice that involves the insertion of thin needles into specific points on the body. While it is commonly used for pain relief, acupuncture has also been found to have a positive impact on stress reduction and overall well-being.

Research has shown that acupuncture can stimulate the release of endorphins, which are natural painkillers and mood enhancers. These endorphins help to reduce stress and promote a sense of relaxation and calmness. By targeting specific acupuncture points, practitioners can help rebalance the body's energy flow and alleviate stress-related symptoms.

When it comes to fertility, acupuncture has gained attention for its potential benefits. Stress has been shown to have a negative impact on fertility, and by reducing stress levels, acupuncture may improve the chances of conception. Studies have suggested that acupuncture can regulate the hypothalamic-pituitary-adrenal (HPA) axis, which plays a crucial role in the body's stress response. By modulating this axis, acupuncture may help restore hormonal balance and enhance reproductive function.

Furthermore, acupuncture can also improve blood circulation to the reproductive organs, which can support the development of healthy follicles and improve the uterine lining. This improved blood flow can also enhance the delivery of nutrients and oxygen to the reproductive system, creating a more favorable environment for conception.

It's important to note that acupuncture should be used as a complementary therapy alongside other fertility treatments or interventions. It is not a standalone solution for infertility. However, when combined with conventional medical approaches, acupuncture can provide a holistic approach to fertility care, addressing both the physical and emotional aspects of the journey.

Overall, acupuncture offers a natural and non-invasive option for stress reduction, which can have a positive impact on fertility outcomes. By promoting relaxation, hormonal balance, and improved blood flow, acupuncture may help individuals and couples navigate the challenges of infertility with greater ease and potentially increase their chances of conceiving.

Herbal Medicine for Stress and Fertility

Herbal Medicine for Stress and Fertility

Herbal medicine has been used for centuries to promote overall well-being and address various health concerns, including stress and fertility. Many herbs and botanicals have adaptogenic properties, meaning they can help the body adapt to and manage stress more effectively.

Additionally, certain herbs have been traditionally used to support reproductive health and enhance fertility.

One popular herb known for its stress-reducing properties is *Ashwagandha*. This adaptogenic herb has been used in Ayurvedic medicine to help the body cope with stress and promote a sense of calm. Research suggests that Ashwagandha may also have positive effects on reproductive health, including improving sperm quality and motility in men and regulating menstrual cycles in women.

Another herb commonly used for stress management and fertility support is *Chasteberry*. Chasteberry, also known as Vitex, is believed to help balance hormones and regulate the menstrual cycle. It may be particularly beneficial for women with irregular periods or hormonal imbalances that can affect fertility.

Maca root is another herb that has gained popularity for its potential benefits in managing stress and supporting fertility. Maca is known as an adaptogen and has been used traditionally to enhance energy, libido, and overall well-being. Some studies suggest that Maca may also have positive effects on sperm quality and reproductive hormone levels.

In addition to these herbs, there are many other botanicals that can be used to manage stress and promote reproductive health. These include *Rhodiola, Ginseng, Licorice root,* and *Passionflower*. It is important to note that while herbal medicine can be a natural and holistic approach to stress management and fertility support, it is always recommended to consult with a qualified healthcare practitioner before incorporating any new herbs or supplements into your routine.

Adaptogenic Herbs for Stress Reduction

Adaptogenic herbs are a natural solution for reducing stress and promoting overall well-being. These powerful plants have been used for centuries in traditional medicine to support the body's ability to adapt to stressors and restore balance. When it comes to fertility, adaptogenic herbs can play a crucial role in reducing stress levels and improving reproductive health.

One popular adaptogenic herb is Ashwagandha, also known as Indian ginseng. Ashwagandha has been shown to reduce cortisol levels, the primary stress hormone, and promote a sense of calmness and relaxation. By reducing stress, Ashwagandha can help regulate hormonal imbalances and enhance fertility outcomes.

Rhodiola rosea is another adaptogenic herb that has been extensively studied for its stress-reducing properties. This herb helps the body adapt to physical and emotional stress, improving energy levels and overall well-being. By reducing stress, Rhodiola rosea can support reproductive health and increase the chances of conception.

Ginseng, particularly Panax ginseng, is also considered an adaptogenic herb with powerful stress-reducing properties. It helps regulate the body's stress response and supports the adrenal glands, which play a crucial role in hormone production. By reducing stress and supporting hormonal balance, ginseng can improve fertility outcomes.

Other adaptogenic herbs that can be beneficial for stress reduction and fertility include Holy basil, Licorice root, and Astragalus. These herbs work by supporting the body's natural stress response and promoting a sense of calmness and relaxation. By reducing stress, they can help optimize reproductive health and increase the chances of successful conception.

It's important to note that while adaptogenic herbs can be beneficial for stress reduction and fertility, it's always recommended to consult with a healthcare professional before incorporating them into your routine. They can provide personalized guidance and ensure that the herbs are safe and appropriate for your specific needs.

Herbal Teas and Infusions for Relaxation

When it comes to reducing stress and promoting relaxation, herbal teas and infusions can be a wonderful addition to your daily routine. These natural beverages not only offer a soothing and calming effect but also provide various health benefits that can positively impact fertility.

One popular herbal tea for relaxation is chamomile tea. Chamomile has been used for centuries as a natural remedy for stress and anxiety. It contains compounds that have a calming effect on the body and can help reduce tension and promote a sense of calmness. By incorporating chamomile tea into your daily routine, you can create a peaceful ritual that allows you to unwind and relax.

In addition to chamomile, other herbal teas and infusions that can help reduce stress and benefit fertility include lavender tea, lemon balm tea, and passionflower tea. Lavender tea is known for its soothing properties and can help calm the mind and body. Lemon balm tea has a mild sedative effect and can promote relaxation and improve sleep quality. Passionflower tea has been traditionally used to alleviate anxiety and promote a sense of calmness.

When preparing herbal teas and infusions, it's important to use high-quality organic herbs and steep them for the recommended amount of time to extract their beneficial properties. You can also experiment with different combinations of herbs to find the flavors and blends that you enjoy the most. Adding a teaspoon of honey or a squeeze of lemon can enhance the taste and provide additional health benefits.

Remember, while herbal teas and infusions can be a helpful tool in managing stress and promoting relaxation, they should not replace professional medical advice or treatment. If you have any concerns about your fertility or are experiencing difficulties conceiving, it's important to consult with a healthcare professional or fertility specialist.

Seeking Professional Help for Stress and Infertility

When dealing with the stress and emotional toll of infertility, it is important to recognize when seeking professional help can be beneficial. Fertility specialists, therapists, and counselors are trained professionals who can provide guidance and support throughout the journey of stress-related fertility issues.

One key aspect to consider is the duration of your struggle with infertility. If you have been actively trying to conceive for a year or more without success, it may be time to consult with a fertility specialist. These medical professionals specialize in diagnosing and treating fertility issues, and they can help identify any underlying medical conditions that may be contributing to your infertility.

Additionally, therapists and counselors can offer valuable emotional support during this challenging time. They can provide a safe space for you to express your feelings, process your emotions, and develop coping strategies to manage stress. Therapy can be particularly beneficial if you are experiencing anxiety, depression, or relationship strain as a result of your infertility journey.

Support groups can also play a vital role in providing guidance and understanding. Connecting with others who are going through similar experiences can offer a sense of community and reduce feelings of isolation. Online communities and local support groups can be excellent resources for finding support and sharing advice.

Remember, seeking professional help does not mean that you have failed or that there is something wrong with you.

Infertility is a complex issue that can impact individuals and couples in various ways. By reaching out to fertility specialists, therapists, and support groups, you are taking proactive steps towards managing stress and improving your overall well-being.

Coping with Infertility-Related Stress

Coping with Infertility-Related Stress

Infertility can be an incredibly stressful and emotional journey for individuals and couples who are struggling to conceive. The constant disappointment, uncertainty, and pressure can take a toll on one's mental and emotional well-being. It is important to acknowledge and address the stress associated with infertility in order to navigate this challenging time with resilience and support.

Here are some coping strategies and support options for individuals and couples experiencing stress due to infertility:

- **Seek emotional support:** Reach out to trusted friends, family members, or support groups who can provide a listening ear and understanding. Sharing your feelings and experiences with others who are going through similar challenges can be incredibly comforting and validating.

- **Consider therapy or counseling:** Professional therapy or counseling can provide a safe space to explore and process the complex emotions that come with infertility. A trained therapist can help individuals and couples develop coping mechanisms, enhance communication skills, and navigate the emotional rollercoaster of fertility struggles.
- **Practice self-care:** Prioritize self-care activities that promote relaxation and stress reduction. Engage in activities that bring you joy and help you unwind, such as taking walks in nature, practicing mindfulness or meditation, indulging in a hobby, or pampering yourself with a massage or spa treatment.
- **Stay informed but set boundaries:** It can be tempting to constantly research and seek information about fertility treatments and options. While it is important to stay informed, it is equally important to set boundaries and give yourself breaks from the constant influx of information. Allow yourself to take time off from thinking about fertility and focus on other aspects of your life.
- **Communicate openly with your partner:** Infertility can strain relationships, so it is crucial to maintain open and honest communication with your partner. Share your

feelings, fears, and hopes with each other, and work together as a team to navigate the challenges. Seek professional help if needed to address any relationship issues that arise due to stress.

Remember, coping with infertility-related stress is a personal journey, and what works for one person may not work for another. It is important to find coping strategies that resonate with you and provide the support you need. Be gentle with yourself and give yourself permission to feel the full range of emotions that come with infertility. Reach out for support when needed, and remember that you are not alone in this journey.

Support Groups and Online Communities

Support groups and online communities can be invaluable resources for individuals and couples facing fertility challenges. Joining these groups provides an opportunity to connect with others who are going through similar experiences, creating a sense of community and understanding. These groups offer a safe space to share emotions, ask questions, and seek advice from others who truly understand the struggles and emotions associated with infertility.

By participating in support groups or online communities, individuals can reduce feelings of isolation and find comfort in knowing that they are not alone in their journey. It can be incredibly reassuring to connect with others who can relate to the ups and downs of fertility treatments, the emotional rollercoaster of trying to conceive, and the challenges of coping with infertility.

Support groups and online communities can also provide valuable information and resources. Members often share their own experiences, tips, and coping strategies, which can be incredibly helpful for those navigating the complex world of fertility. These groups can also serve as a platform for individuals to ask questions and receive guidance from others who have been through similar situations.

Additionally, participating in support groups or online communities can offer a sense of hope and encouragement. Seeing others who have successfully overcome fertility challenges or who are on a similar path can inspire and motivate individuals to keep going and remain optimistic.

In summary, joining support groups and online communities can provide numerous benefits for individuals and couples facing infertility. From connecting with others who understand the journey to gaining valuable information and resources, these communities offer a sense of belonging, reduce feelings of isolation, and provide much-needed support during a challenging time.

Communication and Partner Support

When it comes to managing the stress and emotional challenges of infertility, open communication and partner support play a crucial role. Dealing with fertility issues can be an overwhelming and isolating experience, but having a strong support system can make a significant difference.

Open communication between partners is essential for navigating the emotional journey of infertility. It allows both individuals to express their feelings, fears, and frustrations, creating a safe space for honest conversations. By openly discussing their emotions, couples can better understand each other's perspectives and provide the support and comfort needed during this difficult time.

Additionally, partner support is crucial in managing stress related to infertility. Being there for each other, offering a shoulder to lean on, and actively participating in the fertility journey can strengthen the bond between partners and alleviate some of the stress associated with infertility. Whether it's attending doctor's appointments together, researching treatment options, or simply being present and empathetic, partner support can make the journey feel less daunting.

It's important to remember that infertility affects both partners, and the emotional toll can be overwhelming. By fostering open communication and providing unwavering support, couples can navigate the challenges of infertility together and strengthen their relationship in the process.

Seeking Professional Help for Relationship Issues

When facing infertility, it's important to acknowledge the emotional toll it can take on both individuals and their relationships. The stress and strain of fertility struggles can often lead to tension, communication breakdowns, and feelings of isolation. Seeking professional help through couples therapy or relationship counseling can be a valuable resource for addressing stress-related issues and strengthening the partnership during this challenging time.

Couples therapy or relationship counseling provides a safe and supportive space for partners to explore their emotions, communicate effectively, and develop coping strategies. A trained therapist can help couples navigate the emotional rollercoaster of fertility struggles, offering guidance, support, and tools to manage stress and strengthen their bond.

Through therapy, couples can learn effective communication techniques, gain insight into their individual and shared experiences, and develop strategies to cope with the challenges of infertility. Therapists can also provide guidance on managing expectations, setting boundaries, and finding balance in the midst of fertility treatments.

In addition to addressing stress-related issues, couples therapy or relationship counseling can also help partners navigate the complex decision-making process that often accompanies fertility treatments. It provides a neutral space for partners to explore their options, discuss concerns, and make decisions together.

By seeking professional help for relationship issues, couples can work towards building a stronger foundation and supporting each other through the ups and downs of the fertility journey. It's important to remember that seeking help is not a sign of weakness, but rather a proactive step towards creating a healthier and more resilient partnership.

Self-Care and Stress Reduction

Self-care plays a crucial role in reducing stress levels, improving emotional well-being, and enhancing fertility outcomes. By prioritizing self-care, individuals can create a nurturing environment for their mind and body, which can positively impact their reproductive health. Here are some self-care tips and activities that can help reduce stress and support fertility:

- **Practice relaxation techniques:** Engaging in relaxation techniques such as meditation, deep breathing exercises, or progressive muscle relaxation can help calm the mind and reduce stress levels. These practices promote a sense of relaxation and can improve overall emotional well-being.
- **Engage in regular exercise:** Regular physical activity is not only beneficial for physical health but also plays a significant role in managing stress. Engaging in activities like yoga, walking, or swimming can help release endorphins, which are natural mood boosters.
- **Maintain a balanced diet:** A well-balanced diet rich in nutrients can support overall health and help reduce stress. Incorporating foods that are high in antioxidants, omega-3 fatty acids, and vitamins can provide the body with the

necessary nutrients to combat stress and optimize fertility.

- **Get enough sleep:** Prioritizing quality sleep is essential for managing stress and supporting reproductive health. Aim for 7-8 hours of uninterrupted sleep each night to allow the body to rest and rejuvenate.
- **Engage in hobbies and activities:** Participating in activities that bring joy and relaxation can help reduce stress levels. Whether it's painting, gardening, reading, or listening to music, finding time for hobbies can provide a much-needed break from daily stressors.
- **Connect with loved ones:** Building a support system and maintaining strong relationships can help individuals navigate the emotional challenges of infertility. Regularly connecting with loved ones, whether through phone calls, video chats, or in-person meetings, can provide emotional support and reduce feelings of isolation.
- **Set boundaries and practice self-compassion:** Learning to say no and setting boundaries is essential for self-care. It's important to prioritize personal needs and not feel guilty about taking time for oneself. Practicing self-compassion and treating oneself

with kindness and understanding can also help reduce stress levels.

Remember, self-care is not a luxury but a necessity, especially when dealing with the stress of infertility. By incorporating these self-care tips and activities into daily life, individuals can reduce stress, improve emotional well-being, and enhance their fertility journey.

Frequently Asked Questions

- **1. Can stress affect fertility?**

  Yes, stress can have a significant impact on fertility. Research has shown that high levels of stress can disrupt the reproductive system and interfere with ovulation and sperm production, making it more difficult to conceive.

- **2. How does chronic stress affect women's fertility?**

  Chronic stress can lead to irregular menstrual cycles, hormonal imbalances, and decreased fertility in women. It can also contribute to conditions like polycystic ovary syndrome (PCOS), endometriosis, and uterine fibroids, which can further affect fertility.

- **3. What are the effects of chronic stress on men's fertility?**

Chronic stress can lower sperm count, reduce sperm motility, and increase the risk of erectile dysfunction in men. It can also impact sperm quality, leading to issues with DNA fragmentation, morphology, and overall sperm health.

- **4. How can stress management techniques improve fertility?**

Implementing stress management techniques can help reduce stress levels and improve reproductive health. Techniques such as meditation, yoga, and acupuncture have been shown to be beneficial in reducing stress and enhancing fertility outcomes.

- **5. Can diet and nutrition help reduce stress and improve fertility?**

Yes, maintaining a balanced diet and consuming specific nutrients can help reduce stress and optimize fertility. Certain foods and supplements, such as those rich in antioxidants and omega-3 fatty acids, can support reproductive health and regulate stress hormones.

- **6. Are there any alternative therapies that can help reduce stress and improve fertility?**

Yes, alternative therapies like acupuncture, herbal medicine, and aromatherapy have shown promise in reducing stress and improving fertility. Acupuncture, in particular, has been found to have stress-reducing effects and potential benefits for fertility.

- **7. When should I seek professional help for stress-related fertility issues?**

  If you are experiencing significant stress related to fertility and it is impacting your emotional well-being and ability to cope, it may be beneficial to seek help from fertility specialists, therapists, or counselors. They can provide guidance and support tailored to your specific situation.

- **8. How can I cope with infertility-related stress?**

  Coping with infertility-related stress can be challenging, but there are strategies that can help. Joining support groups or online communities, seeking partner support, practicing self-care, and considering therapy or counseling are all effective ways to manage stress and navigate the emotional journey of infertility.

Have Questions / Comments?

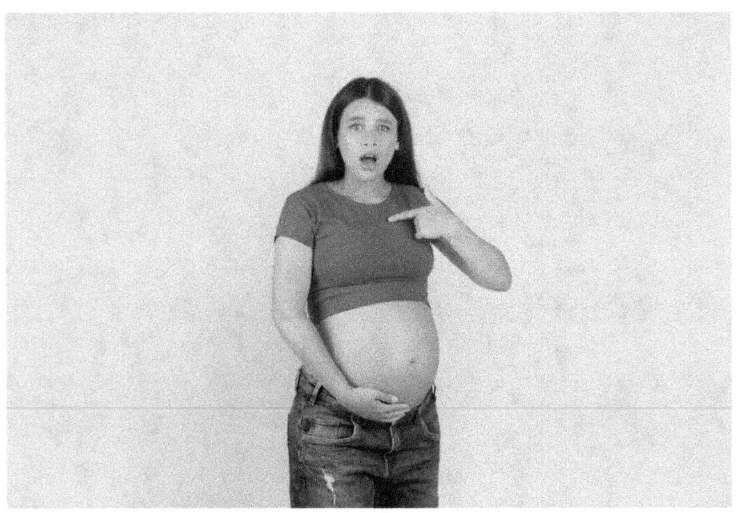

This book was designed to cover as much info as possible but I know I have probably missed something, or some new amazing discovery that has just come out.

If you notice something missing or have a question that I failed to answer, please get in touch and let me know. If I can, I will email you an answer and also update the book so others can also benefit from it.

Thanks For Being Awesome :)

Submit Your Questions / Comments At:

Get How To Be A Super Mom - 100% FREE

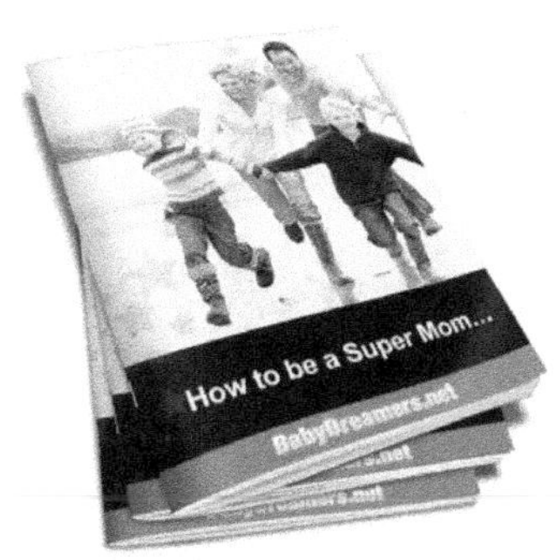

For being one of our amazing readers, we would love to offer you another book we have created, 100% free.

Being a mom is probably the most important job in the world – we've all heard that, and it's true. You're bringing up the next generation of wonderful, intelligent, loving, creative, responsible people.

We all want to be Super Mom and to be everything and do everything, but it this possible?

Being a Super Mom is possible, but you have to learn how to empower yourself to be the kind of Super Mom that you feel you need to be, keeping in mind that the title Super Mom doesn't mean the same thing to everyone.

Get How to be a Super Mom For Free at

BabyDreamers.net

9 798859 334650